ALMIGHTY SESAME

SEEDS:

51 USES OF SESAME

SEED AND ITS SIDE

EFFECTS

Introduction

Sesame plant is a flowering plant belonging to the Pedaliaceae family. These seeds have the highest oil content among all seeds and a delicate, nutty flavor that becomes more pronounced when they are roasted under low temperature for a few minutes. These seeds can be consumed in the raw or dried form, or even as roasted snacks. They are used as an ingredient in several cuisines. Dry roasted sesame seeds are ground with olive into a thin, light brown colored paste, known as 'Tahini', which is a popular Middle Eastern dip. In Europe, they are commonly used in the manufacture of margarine. There are several varieties of sesame seeds depending on the type of cultivar such as white, black and brown seeds White sesame seeds have higher iron content than the black ones and are mostly used as ingredients in food or in the form of oil. Black sesame seeds are more flavorful and have a stronger aroma than white or brown sesame seeds and are preferably used in medicines. They contain 60% more calcium than the white ones. Sesame seeds are tiny, oil-rich seeds that grow in pods on the Sesamum indicum plant.

Unhulled seeds have the outer, edible husk intact, while hulled seeds come without the husk. The hull gives the seeds a golden-brown hue. Hulled seeds have an off-white color but turn brown when roasted. Sesame seeds have many potential health benefits and have been used in folk medicine for thousands of years. They may protect against heart disease, diabetes, and arthritis.

However, you may need to eat significant amounts — a small handful per day — to gain health benefits.

In addition to their culinary uses, these seeds possess nutritive, preventive, and curative properties, which render them usable in traditional medicines. Sesame seed oil is a rich source of phytonutrients such as omega-6 fatty acids, flavonoid phenolic antioxidants, vitamins and dietary fiber. These seeds, thus, offer a variety of benefits. The health benefits of sesame seeds include the following:

51 Health and Nutrition Benefits of Sesame Seeds

1. Good Source of Fiber

Three tablespoons (30 grams) of unhulled sesame seeds provide 3.5 grams of fiber, which is 12% of the Reference Daily Intake (RDI).

Since the average fiber intake in the United States is only half of the RDI, eating sesame seeds regularly could help increase your fiber intake.

Fiber is well known for supporting digestive health. Additionally, growing evidence suggests that fiber may play a role in reducing your risk of heart disease, certain cancers, obesity, and type 2 diabetes.

SUMMARY A 3-tablespoon (30-gram) serving of sesame seeds supplies 12% of the RDI for fiber, which is vital for your digestive health.

2. May Lower Cholesterol and Triglycerides

Some studies suggest that regularly eating sesame seeds may help decrease high cholesterol and triglycerides — which are risk factors for heart disease.

Sesame seeds consist of 15% saturated fat, 41% polyunsaturated fat, and 39% monounsaturated fat

Research indicates that eating more polyunsaturated and monounsaturated fat relative to saturated fat may help lower your cholesterol and reduce heart disease risk.

What's more, sesame seeds contain two types of plant compounds —

lignans and phytosterols — that may also have cholesterol-lowering effects.

When 38 people with high blood lipids ate 5 tablespoons (40 grams) of hulled sesame seeds daily for 2 months, they experienced a 10% reduction in "bad" LDL cholesterol and an 8% reduction in triglycerides compared to the placebo group.

SUMMARY Sesame seeds may help reduce heart disease risk factors, including elevated triglyceride and "bad" LDL cholesterol levels.

3. Nutritious Source of Plant Protein

Sesame seeds supply 5 grams of protein per 3-tablespoon (30-gram) serving.

To maximize protein availability, opt for hulled, roasted sesame seeds. The hulling and roasting processes reduce oxalates and phytates — compounds that hamper your digestion and absorption of protein.

Protein is essential for your health, as it helps build everything from muscles to hormones.

Notably, sesame seeds are low in lysine, an essential amino acid more abundant in animal products. However, vegans and vegetarians can compensate by consuming high-lysine plant proteins — particularly legumes, such as kidney beans and chickpeas.

On the other hand, sesame seeds are high in methionine and cysteine, two amino acids that legumes don't provide in large amounts.

SUMMARY Sesame seeds — particularly hulled ones — are a good source of protein, which is a necessary building block for your body.

4. May Help Lower Blood Pressure

High blood pressure is a major risk factor for heart disease and stroke.

Sesame seeds are high in magnesium, which may help lower blood pressure.

Additionally, lignans, vitamin E, and other antioxidants in sesame seeds may help prevent plaque buildup in your arteries, potentially maintaining healthy blood pressure.

In one study, people with high blood pressure consumed 2.5 grams of powdered, black sesame seeds — a less common variety — in capsule form every day.

At the end of one month, they experienced a 6% decrease in systolic blood pressure — the top number of a blood pressure reading — compared to the placebo group.

SUMMARY Sesame seeds are high in magnesium, which may help lower blood pressure. Additionally, their antioxidants may help prevent plaque buildup.

5. May Support Healthy Bones

Sesame seeds — both unhulled and hulled — are rich in several nutrients that boost bone health, though the calcium is mainly in the hull.

Three tablespoons (30 grams) of sesame seeds boast

However, sesame seeds contain natural compounds called oxalates and phytates, antinutrients that reduce the absorption of these minerals.

To limit these compounds' impact, try soaking, roasting, or sprouting the seeds.

One study found that sprouting reduced phytate and oxalate concentration by about 50% in both hulled and unhulled sesame seeds.

SUMMARY Unhulled sesame seeds are especially rich in nutrients vital to bone health, including calcium. Soaking, roasting, or sprouting sesame seeds can improve absorption of these minerals.

6. May Reduce Inflammation

Sesame seeds may fight inflammation.

Long-term, low-level inflammation may play a role in many chronic conditions, including obesity and cancer, as well as heart and kidney disease

When people with kidney disease ate a mixture of 18 grams of flax seeds and 6 grams each of sesame and pumpkin seeds daily for 3 months, their inflammatory markers dropped 51–79%

However, because this study tested a mixture of seeds, the anti-inflammatory impact of sesame seeds alone is uncertain.

Still, animal studies of sesame seed oil also suggest anti-inflammatory effects This may be due to sesamin, a compound found in sesame seeds and their oil.

SUMMARY Preliminary research suggests that sesame seeds and their oil may have anti-inflammatory properties.

7. Good Source of B Vitamins

Sesame seeds are a good source of certain B vitamins, which are distributed both in the hull and seed

Removing the hull may either concentrate or remove some of the B vitamins. B vitamins are essential for many bodily processes, including proper cell function and metabolism

SUMMARY Sesame seeds are a good source of thiamine, niacin, and vitamin B6, which are necessary for proper cellular function and metabolism.

To help you be well, we'll send you honest talk about women's bodies, and beauty, nutrition, and fitness advice.

8. May Aid Blood Cell Formation

To make red blood cells, your body needs several nutrients — including ones found in sesame seeds. SUMMARY Sesame seeds supply iron, copper, and vitamin B6, which are needed for blood cell formation and function.

9. May Aid Blood Sugar Control

Sesame seeds are low in carbs while high in protein and healthy fats — all of which may support blood sugar control.

Additionally, these seeds contain pinoresinol, a compound that may help regulate blood sugar by inhibiting the action of the digestive enzyme maltase.

Maltase breaks down the sugar maltose, which is used as a sweetener for some food products. It's also produced in your gut from the digestion of starchy foods like bread and pasta.

If pinoresinol inhibits your digestion of maltose, this may result in lower blood sugar levels. However, human studies are needed.

SUMMARY Sesame seeds may aid blood sugar control because they're low in carbs and high in quality protein and healthy fats. What's more, they contain a plant compound that may help in this regard.

10. Rich in Antioxidants

Animal and human studies suggest that consuming sesame seeds may increase the overall amount of antioxidant activity in your blood

The lignans in sesame seeds function as antioxidants, which help fight oxidative stress — a chemical reaction that may damage your cells and increase your risk of many chronic diseases.

Additionally, sesame seeds contain a form of vitamin E called gamma-tocopherol, an antioxidant that may be especially protective against heart disease.

SUMMARY Plant compounds and vitamin E in sesame seeds function as antioxidants, which combat oxidative stress in your body.

11. May Support Your Immune System

Sesame seeds are a good source of several nutrients crucial for your immune system, including zinc, selenium, copper, iron, vitamin B6, and vitamin E.

For example, your body needs zinc to develop and activate certain white blood cells that recognize and attack invading microbes.

Keep in mind that even mild to moderate zinc deficiency can impair immune system activity.

Sesame seeds supply about 20% of the RDI for zinc in a 3-tablespoon (30-gram) serving.

SUMMARY Sesame seeds are a good source of several nutrients that are important for immune system function, including zinc, selenium, copper, iron, vitamin B6, and vitamin E.

12. May Soothe Arthritic Knee Pain

Osteoarthritis is the most common cause of joint pain and frequently affects the knees.

Several factors may play a role in arthritis, including inflammation and oxidative damage to the cartilage that cushions joints.

Sesamin, a compound in sesame seeds, has anti-inflammatory and antioxidant effects that may protect your cartilage.

In a 2-month study, people with knee arthritis ate 5 tablespoons (40 grams) of sesame seed powder daily alongside drug therapy. They experienced a 63% decrease in knee pain compared to only a 22% decrease for the group on drug therapy alone.

Additionally, the sesame seed group showed greater improvement in a simple mobility test and larger reductions in certain inflammatory markers compared to the control group.

SUMMARY Sesamin, a compound in sesame seeds, may help reduce joint pain and support mobility in arthritis of the knee.

13. May Support Thyroid Health

Sesame seeds are a good source of selenium, supplying 18% of the RDI in both unhulled and hulled seeds.

Your thyroid gland contains the highest concentration of selenium of any organ in your body. This mineral plays a vital role in making thyroid hormones. In addition, sesame seeds are a good source of iron, copper, zinc, and vitamin B6, which also support the production of thyroid hormones and aid thyroid health.

SUMMARY Sesame seeds are good sources of nutrients — such as selenium, iron, copper, zinc, and vitamin B6 — that support thyroid health.

14. May Aid Hormone Balance During Menopause

Sesame seeds contain phytoestrogens, plant compounds that are similar to the hormone estrogen.

Therefore, sesame seeds might be beneficial for women when estrogen levels drop during menopause. For example, phytoestrogens may help counteract hot flashes and other symptoms of low estrogen. What's more, these compounds may decrease your risk of certain diseases — such as breast cancer — during menopause. However, further research is needed.

SUMMARY Phytoestrogens are compounds found in sesame seeds that may benefit women who are undergoing menopause.

15. Easy to Add to Your Diet

Sesame seeds can give a nutty flavor and subtle crunch to many dishes.

To enhance the flavor and nutrient availability of sesame seeds, roast them at 350°F (180°C) for a few minutes, stirring periodically, until they reach a light, golden brown.

Try adding sesame seeds to:

• stir-fries

- steamed broccoli

- hot or cold cereal

- granola and granola bars

- bread and muffins

- crackers

- yogurt

- smoothies

- salads

- salad dressing

- hummus

- garnishes

Additionally, you can use sesame seed butter — also known as tahini — in place of peanut butter or hummus.

Ground sesame seeds — called sesame flour or sesame seed meal — can be used in baking, smoothies, fish batter, and more.

However, sesame allergies have become more prevalent, so you may need to take caution when cooking for groups.

SUMMARY Sesame seeds can perk up many dishes, including salads, granola, baked goods, and stir-fries.

Tahini and sesame flour are other products made out of sesame seeds.

16. High Protein Vegetarian Diet

Sesame seeds are a good source of dietary protein, with high-quality amino acids making up 20% of the seed. Thus, they are perfect to form part of a high-protein vegetarian diet. Just sprinkle them over your salads, veggies, and noodles.

17. Prevent Diabetes

Sesame seeds contain magnesium and other nutrients that have been shown to combat diabetes. The usage of sesame seed oil as the sole edible oil has been found to be effective in lowering the blood pressure and plasma glucose in hypersensitive diabetics.

18. Cure Anemia

Sesame seeds, particularly the black ones, are rich in iron. Hence, they are highly recommended for those suffering from anemia and weakness.

19. Cardiovascular Health

- Sesame seed oil prevents atherosclerotic lesions and hence, is beneficial for the heart health.

• They contain an antioxidant and anti-inflammatory compound called sesamol that also exhibits anti-atherogenic properties, thus improving the cardiovascular health.

• Sesame seeds are high in the monounsaturated fatty acid, oleic acid, which helps in lowering the bad cholesterol and increasing the good cholesterol in the body. This prevents the risk of coronary artery disease and strokes.

20. Anti-Cancer Properties

Sesame seeds contain magnesium which has anti-cancer properties. They also contain an anti-cancer compound called phytate. Sesame seeds have proven to be effective in reducing the risk of colorectal tumors, thus preventing colorectal cancer.

21. Digestive Health

Sesame seeds support a healthy digestive system and colon as they are rich in fiber. This high fiber content helps in smooth functioning of the intestine, thus facilitating waste disposal and relieving constipation.

22. Relief From Rheumatoid Arthritis

Sesame seeds contain copper, a mineral that is vital for antioxidant enzyme systems, thus reducing the pain and swelling associated with arthritis. Besides, this mineral provides strength to the blood vessels, bones, and joints.

23. Respiratory Health

Magnesium contained in sesame seeds prevents asthma and other respiratory disorders by preventing airway spasms.

24. Protection From Radiation Damage

Sesamol, found in sesame seeds and sesame oil, has been found to prevent the DNA from being damaged by radiation. It also prevents damage to the intestines and the spleen.

25. Bone Health

Sesame seeds contain zinc that boosts the bone mineral density and the bone health. The deficiency of this mineral can cause osteoporosis in the hip and spine area. Sesame seeds are a great source of calcium, a trace mineral that is vital to bone health.

26. Oral Health

Sesame seeds and sesame seed oil help in boosting the oral health by removing dental plaque and whitening your teeth. Oil pulling, i.e. swishing your sesame seed oil in your mouth, can reduce the amount of streptococcus mutants in both the teeth and the mouth saliva and boost the overall health

27. Nullify The Effects Of Alcohol

Sesame seeds help the liver to decompose the harmful effects of alcohol as well as other substances that generate poisoning in the body.

28. Treatment Of Anxiety

• Sesame seeds contain several nutrients that have stress-relieving properties.

• Minerals like magnesium and calcium act as an antispasmodic by regulating the muscle function i.e. contraction and relaxation.

- Thiamin (vitamin B1) has calming properties that aid in proper nerve functioning. The deficiency of this vitamin can lead to muscle spasms, moodiness, and depression.

- Tryptophan is an essential amino acid that is involved in the production of serotonin, a neurotransmitter that reduces pain and regulates the sleep pattern and mood. The inadequacy of serotonin production and transmission in the brain can result in anxiety and depression.

29. Lower Cholesterol

• Black sesame seeds benefit in lowering the cholesterol levels. They contain two substances called sesamin and sesamolin, which belong to a group of fibers called lignans. Lignans have a cholesterol lowering effect as they are rich in dietary fiber.

• Black sesame seeds also contain plant compounds called phytosterols which have a structure similar to that of cholesterol. Their consumption not only decreases the blood cholesterol levels, but also reduces the risk of developing certain types of cancer.

- Sesame seeds have the highest phytosterol content of all seeds and nuts.

30. Eye Health

- According to traditional Chinese medicine, there is a strong relationship between the internal organs and external parts such as the eyes and the liver.

The liver stores blood and since a certain branch of the liver channel goes to the eyes, the liver can also send blood to the eyes to support their functioning.

• Black sesame seeds are beneficial for the liver as they increase the liver blood, thereby nourishing the eyes. Their therapeutic effects help in treating blurred vision and tired, dry eyes.

31. Nourish The Organs

Black sesame seeds have been found to increase energy, nourish the brain and slow down aging. The regular consumption of black sesame seeds can help reduce the symptoms of backache, painful or tight and stiff joints, and weakness in the joints.

32. Blood Pressure Reduction

Nowadays hypertension is a common health problem among women and men from various age groups. Studies have indicated that using this oil can help reduce hypertension. The magnesium in this oil helps reduce blood pressure.

The extensive range of minerals and vitamins in this oil help boost your immunity. Its antioxidants and these nutrients help the body fight cancer causing elements in a better way. The phytates present in these seeds are known for their cancer preventing properties too.

33. Anti-Inflammatory Effects

Using black sesame seed oil, either topically or by consumption, can help reduce ailments and conditions caused by inflammation. The high amount of copper in this oil helps the users cope better with inflammation caused conditions affecting the body joints.

Skin Benefits Of Sesame Seeds

Sesame is rich in powerful antioxidants and possesses antibacterial and antiviral properties. It offers several benefits to your skin by bringing blood and nourishment. The oil extracted from sesame seeds is rich in omega-6, calcium, magnesium, phosphorus, iron, and vitamins B and E which have been used as products of beautification. Let us learn how sesame seeds are beneficial for the skin.

34. Healing Properties

Sesame seed oil is a natural anti-inflammatory agent and has excellent healing properties. Its antibacterial properties help to get rid of skin pathogens like staphylococcus and streptococcus as well as common skin fungi such as athlete's foot fungus. Sesame seed oil mixed with warm water can control vaginal yeast infections.

35. Treatment Of Sunburns

When used after the exposure to the wind or the sun, sesame seed oil can treat suntans. It prevents the harmful ultraviolet rays of the sun from damaging your skin, thus preventing the appearance of wrinkles and pigmentation. The regular usage of this oil significantly reduces the risk of skin cancer and prevents the skin from the effects of chlorine in swimming pool water.

36. Skin Detoxifier

The antioxidants contained in sesame seed oil help in detoxifying your skin When applied on the skin, the molecules of this oil attract oil-soluble toxins that can be washed away with hot water and soap.

• Mix half a cup of sesame seed oil with half a cup of apple cider vinegar and a quarter cup of water.

• This should be applied every night after splashing your face with water.

You should include sesame seed oil in your beauty regime.

37. Suitable For Babies

Baby skin, particularly the area covered with diapers, often gets rashes due to the acidity of body wastes. Sesame seed oil protects their tender skin against these rashes. Applying it to the nose and ears provides protection against common skin pathogens. It also combats dryness of skin.

38. Glowing Skin

• Sesame seed oil can provide you with glowing skin. It maintains skin flexibility by keeping it soft and supple, and heals the areas of mild cuts, scrapes and abrasions.

• It helps tighten the facial skin, particularly the area around the nose, and controls the enlargement of pores.

• It also controls eruptions and neutralizes the poisons which develop on the surface and in the pores.

• You can also try a facial for glowing skin.

- Massage your face thoroughly with sesame seed oil and scrub your face with rice or besan powder before washing off with warm water.

- Later, splash your face with cold water to close the pores.

39. Treatment Of Cracked Heels

If you have cracked heels or sore feet, you can apply sesame seed oil every night before going to bed and cover your feet with cotton socks. This should be done for a couple of days to get soft and supple feet.

Hair Benefits Of Sesame Seeds

Sesame seeds are packed with vitamins, nutrients and minerals that are vital for the maintenance of a healthy scalp and hair. Just like the skin, sesame seed oil has beneficial effects on your scalp, thus combating various scalp problems. The benefits of sesame seeds for the scalp are as follows.

40. Encourage Hair Growth

Sesame seeds contain essential fatty acids such as omega-3, omega-6 and omega-9 which promote hair growth. Sesame seed oil stimulates hair growth by nourishing, conditioning, and promoting a healthy scalp. The regular massage with warm sesame oil penetrates your scalp, thus increasing the blood circulation. It is comparable to a liquid vitamin that feeds your hair roots and shafts

41. Prevention Of Scalp Problems

Sesame seeds are rich in replenishing vitamins, minerals and nutrients that are vital for a healthy scalp. Massaging your scalp with sesame seed oil combats dryness, flakiness and clogged pores that cause hair thinning and hair loss. Besides, its antifungal, antibacterial and anti-inflammatory properties help in treating scalp infections and dandruff and soothing an irritated scalp.

42. Natural Sunscreen

Sesame seed oil acts as a natural sunscreen for your hair by protecting it from the damaging effects of the sun's ultraviolet rays and pollution.

43. Deep Conditioning

Sesame seed oil acts as a deep conditioning treatment for dry, damaged hair, split ends or chemically treated hair. It restores the lost moisture and strengthens the hair shaft, enabling dull and brittle hair to regain its shine, bounce, elasticity and softness.

44. Hair Darkening Qualities

Sesame seed oil is known for its hair darkening qualities that make it effective for people suffering from premature graying of hair. It can be used with carrier oils like olive or almond oil to reap the maximum benefits.

45. High in Fiber

Sesame seeds are packed with a significant amount of fiber, an important element in healthy digestion. It can reduce conditions like constipation and diarrhea, while simultaneously protecting the health of your colon and reducing the risk of gastrointestinal diseases. Fiber also works beneficially for your heart, by scraping out dangerous LDL cholesterol from arteries and blood vessels, thereby acting as a protecting agent against atherosclerosis, heart attacks, and strokes.

46. Manages Diabetes

Sesame seeds contain magnesium, an important mineral, that aids in reducing the chances of type-2 diabetes. It also regulates blood pressure and helps improve insulin sensitivity. Furthermore, it has been shown that sesame seed oil positively affects the impact of various medications like glibenclamide in patients suffering from type-2 diabetes. It improves the medication's functionality and regulates the insulin and glucose levels in the body. This process helps to manage the symptoms of diabetes, as per a research published in the journal

47. Boosts Bone Health

Sesame is the richest source of most of the inorganic nutrients, says a report published in the Journal of the American Oil Chemists Society. The impressive levels of essential minerals like zinc, calcium, and phosphorus can be a major boost for your bone health. These minerals are integral parts in creating new bone matter and strengthening and repairing bones weakened by injury or the onset of debilitating bone conditions like

48. Improves Oral Health

Perhaps the most notable effects of sesame seeds are its powerful effects on oral health. Oil pulling with sesame seed oil can have a strong antibacterial and astringent effect on all aspects of oral health. It is also closely associated with reducing the presence of the Streptococcus bacteria, a common bacteria that can wreak havoc on your oral cavities and other parts of your body.

49. Increases Fertility in Men

Sesame seeds, when added to the diet of men, improves sperm quality and increases male fertility. A 2013 study published in the Journal of Research in Medical Sciences showed that 25 infertile men, aged between 27 and 40 years, were given sesame seeds for three months. They showed a significant improvement in their sperm count and motility.

50. Reduces Inflammation

The high content of copper in sesame seeds helps in reducing inflammation in joints, bones, and muscles, thereby contributing to preventing the associated pain of arthritis. Furthermore, copper is an essential mineral for strengthening blood vessels, bones, and joints. Finally, copper is necessary for the proper uptake of iron, a key component of hemoglobin. Therefore, proper copper content in the body maximizes circulation and ensures that the organ systems of the entire body receive enough oxygen to function properly.

51. Boosts Metabolic Function

Sesame seeds contain a high amount of protein, which gets broken down and reassembled from its parts into usable proteins for the human body. This adds to overall strength, healthy cellular growth, mobility, energy levels, and a boosted metabolic function. This is confirmed in research published in the Journal of Agricultural and Food Chemistry.

Eating Sesame Seeds

Sesame seeds can be used in a variety of ways. They can be consumed in the following ways:

• Sprinkled as a topping on salads or stews

• Mixed into bread

• Ground into thin paste-like tahini

• Blended into a powder and mixed with various smoothies

Sesame oil is also very popular and potent for natural health remedies, ranging from topical applications on the body to using the oil as an anti-inflammatory substance.

How to eat black sesame seeds?

You should soak the black sesame seeds in water overnight to make them easily digestible. Then, you can sprinkle them on your salads, in your yogurt, or even blend them into a smoothie.

Side Effects

The side effects of sesame seeds occur only when they are consumed in very large amounts. These include:

- Allergy: Excessive consumption of sesame seeds can irritate the stomach and colon.

- Blood sugar levels: People who are diabetic need to be careful, as sesame seeds can increase blood sugar levels. However, more research studies are required to support this claim.

Note: Sesame seeds are not nuts, although many people treat them that way. The reason for this is the presence of similar allergenic chemicals and proteins, which are also found in nuts. Therefore, if you are allergic to some types of nuts, it would

be wise to speak to your doctor about

sesame seeds.

THE BOTTOM LINE

Sesame seeds are a good source of healthy fats, protein, B vitamins, minerals, fiber, antioxidants, and other beneficial plant compounds.

Regularly eating substantial portions of these seeds — not just an occasional sprinkling on a burger bun — may aid blood sugar control, combat arthritis pain, and lower cholesterol.

To optimize your nutrient intake, you can eat sesame seeds soaked, roasted, or sprouted.

www.ingramcontent.com/pod-product-compliance
Lightning Source LLC
Chambersburg PA
CBHW050053260726
48658CB00005B/1924